THE SUPER-NATURAL
PLANT-BASED COOKBOOK

*The Best 50 Plant-Based Recipes to
Celebrate the Natural World*

Botanika Green Way

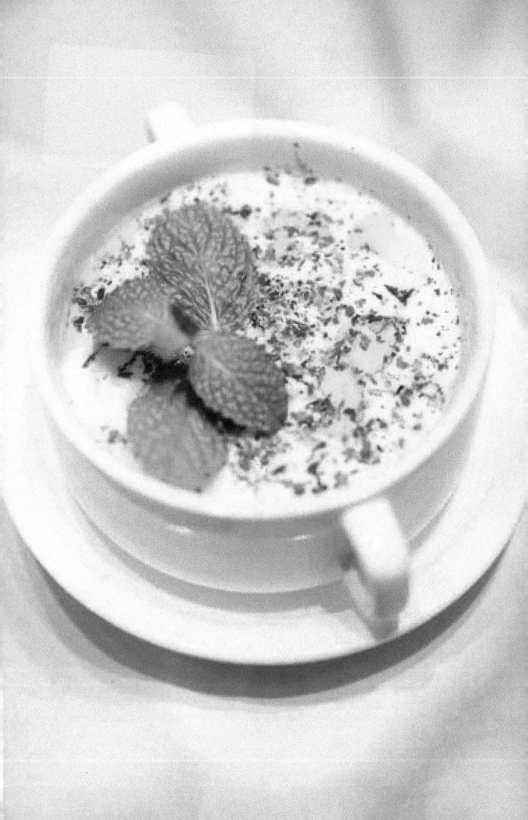

Table of Contents

INTRODUCTION

A plant-based diet is a diet based primarily on whole plant foods. Hence, it excludes animal-sourced foods, hydrogenated oils, refined sugars, and processed foods. A whole food plant-based diet does not consist solely of fruits and vegetables. It includes unprocessed or barely processed oils with healthy fats like extra-virgin olive oil, whole grains, legumes, seeds, and nuts, as well as herbs and spices.

What is the Plant-Based Diet?

The plant-based diet may seem similar to a vegetarian or vegan diet, but it is neither. It's not a diet but a healthy lifestyle. It uses food from plants, and it excludes processed foods like white rice and added sugars, which are allowed in vegan and vegetarian diets.

A plant-based diet is not a diet; it's a healthy way of life

The secret to a healthy diet is simpler than you ever thought! When following a plant-based dietary regimen, you should focus on plant-based foods and avoid animal-sourced food. Whether you are already following a vegan diet or are considering trying this lifestyle, this plant-based, budget-friendly food list makes your grocery shopping easy to manage.

- **VEGETABLES**

Try to include different types of vegetables in your diet from above-ground vegetables to root vegetables, which grow underground.

- **FRUITS**

Choose affordable fruits that are in season. Add frozen fruit to your grocery list since they are just as nutritious as fresh produce. They can be used in smoothies, toppings, compotes, or preserves. On the other hand, dried fruit generally contains a lot of antioxidants, especially polyphenols. It has been proven that eating dried fruits can prevent heart disease and some types of cancer.

- **NUTS & SEEDS**

Nuts and seeds offer different dietary benefits. They do not only ensure essential nutrients but are also offer a variety of flavors. This "ready to eat" food is a perfect snack with dried fruits and trail mix, essential vegan foods to stockpile for an emergency.

- **RICE & GRAINS**

Rice and grains are versatile and easy to incorporate into your diet. Leftovers reheat wonderfully and can be served at any time of the day, turning simple and inexpensive ingredients into a full-fledged meal. You can also make healthy nut butters such as tahini or peanut butter.

- **BEANS & LEGUMES**

Legumes and beans are highly affordable, and there's no end to the variety of tasty dishes you can cook with them. These humble but powerful foods are packed with vitamins, minerals, protein, and dietary fiber. In addition to being super-healthy and versatile, legumes pair very well with other proteins, vegetables, and grains.

- **HEALTHY FATS**

Don't underestimate the importance of quality fats in cooking. Coconut oil, olive oil, and avocado are always good to have on hand.

- **NON-DAIRY PRODUCTS**

Using a plant-based cheese or milk lends flavor, texture, and nutrition to your meals. You can find fantastic products on the market, and this book has many wonderful recipes for feta, vegan ricotta, and plant-based milk.

- **HERBS, SPICES & CONDIMENTS**

A handful of fresh herbs will add that little something extra to your soups, stews, dips, or casseroles. Condiments such as mustard, ketchup, vegan mayonnaise, and plant-based sauces can be used in salads, casseroles, and spreads. Choosing their distinctive flavors to complement vegetables, grains and legumes will help you to make the most of your vegan dishes. Herbs and spices are naturally plant-based, but play it safe and look for a label that says *Vegan-friendly*.

- **BAKING GOODS & CANNED GOODS**

These vegan essentials include all types of flour, baking powder, baking soda, and yeast. Further, cocoa powder, vegan chocolate, and sweeteners are good to have on hand. As for the healthy vegan sweeteners, opt for fresh or dried fruits, agave syrup, maple syrup, and stevia. When it comes to canned goods, stock your pantry with cooking essentials such as tomato, sauerkraut, pickles, low sodium chickpeas and beans, coconut milk, green chilies, pumpkin puree, tomato sauce, low sodium corn, and artichoke hearts. Thus, if you want to make sure you have nutritious, delicious, and quality meals for you and your family, having a vegan pantry is halfway there.

Why You Ought to Reduce Your Intake of Processed and Animal-Based Foods

You have heard over and over that processed food has adverse effects on your health. You might have also been told repeatedly to stay away from foods with lots of preservatives. However, you may have never heard any genuine or concrete facts about why these foods are unsafe. Consequently, let us properly dissect it to help you properly comprehend why you ought to stay away from these offenders.

- **They have massive habit-forming characteristics**

Humans have a predisposition toward being addicted to some specific foods; however, the reality is that the fault is not wholly ours.

Every one of the unhealthy treats we relish now and then triggers a dopamine release. This creates a pleasurable effect in our brain, but the excitement is usually short-lived. The discharged dopamine gradually causes an attachment, and this is the reason some people consistently go back to eat certain unhealthy foods even when they know they're unhealthy and unnecessary. You can get rid of this by avoiding the temptation completely.

- **They are sugar-laden and heavy in glucose-fructose syrup**

Animal-based and processed foods are laden with refined sugars and glucose-fructose syrup, which has almost no nutritional value. An ever-increasing number of studies are affirming what several people presumed from the start: that genetically modified foods bring about inflammatory bowel disease, which consequently makes it increasingly difficult for the body to assimilate essential nutrients. The disadvantages that result from your body being unable to assimilate essential nutrients from consumed foods rightly cannot be overemphasized.

Processed and animal-based food products contain plenteous amounts of refined carbohydrates. Indeed, your body requires carbohydrates to give it energy to function.

In any case, refining carbs dispenses with the fundamental supplements in the way that refining entire grains disposes of the whole grain part. What remains in the wake of refining is what's considered empty carbs or empty calories. These can negatively affect the metabolic system in your body by sharply increasing your blood sugar and insulin levels.

- **They contain lots of synthetic ingredients**

When your body takes in non-natural ingredients, it regards them as a foreign substance and a health threat. It isn't accustomed to identifying synthetic compounds like sucralose or synthesized sugars. Hence, in defense of your health against this foreign "aggressor," your body does what it's programmed to do to safeguard your health: It sets off an immune reaction to tackle this "enemy" compound, which indirectly weakens your body's general disease alertness, making you susceptible to illnesses. The energy expended by your body in triggering your immune system could be better utilized somewhere else.

- **They contain constituent elements that set off a sensation in your body**

A part of processed and animal-based foods contains compounds like glucose-fructose syrup, monosodium glutamate, and specific food dyes that can trigger some addictions. They teach your body to receive a benefit whenever you consume them. Monosodium glutamate, for example, is added to many store-bought baked foods. This additive slowly conditions your palate to relish and crave the taste.

- **This reward-centric arrangement makes you crave it increasingly, which ends up exposing you to the danger of over-consuming calories**

For animal protein, usually, the expression "subpar" is used to allude to plant proteins since they generally have lower levels of essential amino acids as against animal-sourced protein. Nevertheless, what the vast majority don't know is that large amounts of essential amino acids can prove detrimental to your health. Let me break it down further for you.

- **Animal-sourced protein has no fiber**

In their pursuit to consume animal protein, the vast majority wind up dislodging the plant protein that was previously available in their body. Replacing the plant proteins with its animal variant is harmful because, in contrast to plant protein, animal proteins typically are deficient in fiber, phyto-nutrients, and antioxidant properties. Fiber insufficiency is a regular feature across various regions and societies on the planet. In America, for example, according to the National Academy of Medicine, the typical adult takes in roughly 15 grams of dietary fiber daily rather than the recommended daily quantity of 25 to 30 grams. A deficiency in dietary fiber often leads to a heightened risk of breast and colorectal cancers, in addition to constipation, inflammatory bowel disease, and cardiovascular disease.

- **Animal protein brings about an upsurge in phosphorus levels in the body**

Animal protein has significant levels of phosphorus. Our bodies stabilize these plenteous amounts of phosphorus by producing and discharging a hormone known as fibroblast growth factor 23 (FGF23). Studies have shown that this hormone is dangerous to our veins. FGF23 also causes asymmetrical expansion of heart muscles—a determinant for congestive heart failure and even mortality in some advanced cases.

Having discussed the many problems associated with animal protein, it becomes more apt to replace its "high quality" perception with the tag "highly hazardous." In contrast to caffeine, which has a withdrawal effect if it's discontinued abruptly, you can stop taking processed and animal-based foods right away without any withdrawals. Possibly the only thing that you'll give up is the ease of some meals taking little to no time to prepare.

Health Benefits of the Plant-Based Diet

Plant-based eating is one of the healthiest diets in the world. It should include plenty of fresh products, whole grains, legumes, and healthy fats such as seeds and nuts, which are rich in antioxidants, minerals, vitamins, and dietary fiber.

Scientific research has shown that higher use of plant-based foods is connected to a lower risk of death from conditions such as cardiovascular disease, diabetes, hypertension, and obesity. Vegan eating relies heavily on healthy staples, avoiding animal products. Animal products contain much more fat than plant-based foods; it's not a shocker that studies have shown that meat-eaters have nine times the obesity rate of vegans.

This leads us to the next point, one of the greatest benefits of the vegan diet: weight loss. While many people choose to live a vegan life for ethical reasons, the diet itself can help you achieve your weight loss goals. If you're struggling to shift pounds, you may want to consider trying a plant-based diet. How exactly? As a vegan, you will reduce the number of high-calorie foods such as full-fat dairy products, fatty fish, pork, and other cholesterol-containing foods such as eggs. Try replacing such foods with high-fiber and protein-rich alternatives that will keep you fuller longer. The key is focusing on nutrient-dense, clean and natural foods and avoiding empty calories such as sugar, saturated fats, and highly processed foods. Here are a few tricks that help me maintain my weight on the vegan diet. I eat vegetables as a main course; I consume good fats in moderation (good fats such as olive oil do not make you fat); I exercise regularly and cook at home. Plant foods are an excellent source of many nutrients that boost the body's metabolism in many ways. They are easy to digest thanks to their rich content of antioxidants.

- **Reduced Risk of Heart Diseases**

Processed and animal foods are responsible for much heart disease. A whole foods plant-based diet is better at nourishing the body with essential nutrients while improving the heart's function to produce and transport blood to and from the various body parts.

- **Prevents and Heals Diabetes**

Plant-based foods are excellent at reducing high blood sugar. Many studies comparing a vegetarian and vegan diet to a regular meat-filled diet proved that dieting with more plant foods reduced the risk of diabetes by 50 percent.

- **Improved Cognitive Incline**

Fruits and vegetables are excellent for cleansing and boosting metabolism. They release high numbers of plant compounds and antioxidants that slow or prevent cognitive decline. On a plant-based diet, the brain is boosted with sustainable energy, promoting sharp memory, language, thinking, and judgment abilities.

- **Quick Weight Loss**

A high animal food diet is known to drive weight gain. Switching to a plant-based diet helps the body shed fat walls easily, which quickly drives weight loss.

BREAKFAST

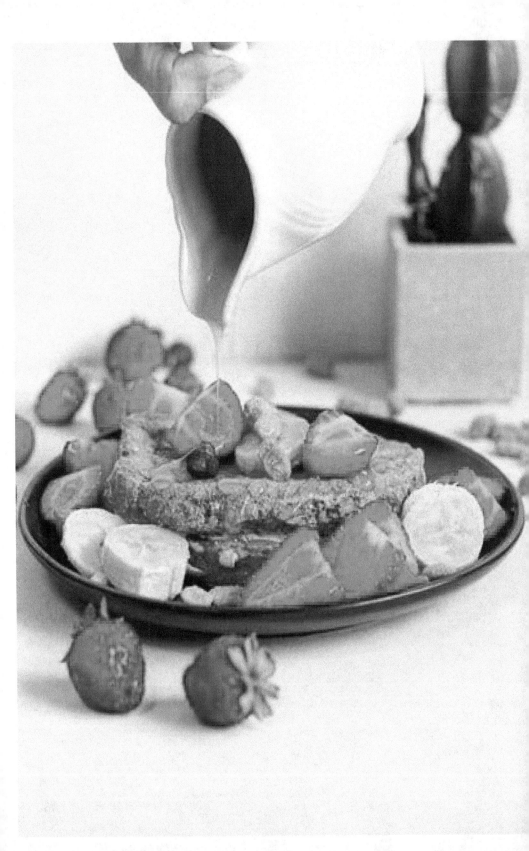

Classic French Toasts

4 Servings

Preparation Time: 16 minutes

Ingredients

- 4 tbsps Flaxseed
- 2 tbsps Coconut flour
- 2 tbsps Almond flour
- 1 ½ tsps Baking powder
- A pinch of Salt
- 2 tbsps Coconut cream
- 2 tbsps Coconut milk whipping cream
- ½ tsp Cinnamon powder
- 1 tsp Plant butter
- 2 tbsps Plant butter

Directions

- For the vegan "flax egg," whisk flax seed powder and 12 tbsps water in two separate bowls and leave to soak for 5 minutes.

- Grease a glass dish (for the microwave) with 1 tsp plant butter.

- In another bowl, mix coconut flour, almond flour, baking powder, and salt.

- When the flaxseed egg is ready, whisk one portion with the coconut cream and add the mixture to the dry ingredients.

- Continue whisking until the mixture is smooth with no lumps.

- Pour the dough into the glass dish and microwave for 2 minutes or until the bread's middle part is done.

- Take out and allow the bread to cool. Remove the bread and slice in half. Return to the glass dish.

- Whisk the remaining vegan "flax egg" with the coconut milk whipping cream until well combined.

- Pour the mixture over the bread slices and leave to soak. Turn the bread a few times to soak in as much of the batter.

- Melt 2 tbsps of the plant butter in a frying pan and fry the bread slices on both sides.

- Transfer to a serving plate, sprinkle with cinnamon powder and serve.

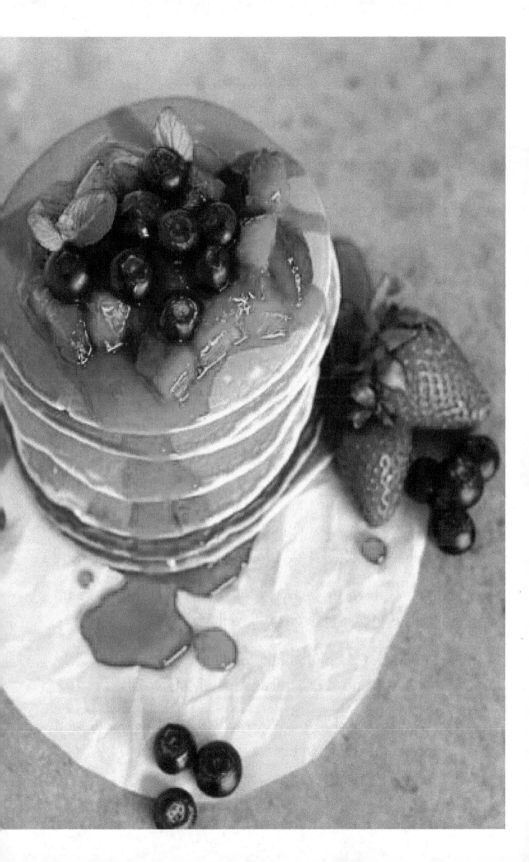

Creamy Sesame Bread

8 Servings

Preparation Time: 40 minutes

Ingredients

- 4 tbsps Flax seed powder
- 4 tbsps Sesame oil + for brushing
- 1 cup Coconut flour
- 2 tbsps Psyllium husk powder
- 1 tsp Salt
- 1 tsp Baking powder
- 2/3 cup Cashew cream cheese
- 1 tbsp Sesame seeds

Directions

- In a bowl, mix the flax seed powder with 1 ½ cups water until smoothly combined and set aside to soak for 5 minutes. Preheat oven to 400°F.

- When the vegan "flax egg" is ready, beat in the cream cheese and sesame oil until well mixed.

- Mix in the coconut flour, psyllium husk powder, salt, and baking powder until adequately blended.

- Oil a 9 x 5 inches baking tray with cooking spray, and spread the dough in the tray.

- Allow the mixture to stand for 5 minutes, and then brush with some sesame oil.

- Sprinkle with the sesame seeds and bake the dough for 30 minutes or until golden brown on top and set within.

- Take out the bread and allow cooling for a few minutes. Slice and serve.

Mixed Seeds Bread

8 Servings

Preparation Time: 55 minutes

Ingredients

- 3 tbsps ground Flax seeds
- 5 tbsps Sesame seeds
- ½ cup Chia seeds
- 1 tsp ground Caraway seeds
- 1 tsp Hemp seeds
- ¼ cup Psyllium husk powder
- 1 tsp Salt
- 2/3 cup Cashew cream cheese
- ½ cup melted Coconut oil
- ¾ cup coconut cream
- ¾ cup coconut flour
- 1 cup almond flour
- 3 tsps baking powder
- 1 tbsp poppy seeds

Directions

- Preheat oven to 350°F and line a loaf pan with parchment paper.

- For the vegan "flax egg," whisk flax seed powder with ½ cup of water and let the mixture sit to soak for 5 minutes.

- In a bowl, mix the coconut flour, almond flour, baking powder, sesame seeds, chia seeds, ground caraway seeds, hemp seeds, psyllium husk powder, and salt.

- In another bowl, use an electric hand mixer to whisk the cream cheese, coconut oil, coconut whipping cream, and vegan "flax egg."

- Add the liquid ingredients into the dry ingredients, and continue whisking with the hand mixer until a dough forms.

- Transfer the dough to the loaf pan, sprinkle with poppy seeds, and bake in the oven for 45 minutes or until a knife inserted into the bread comes out clean.

- Remove the parchment paper with the bread, and allow cooling on a rack.

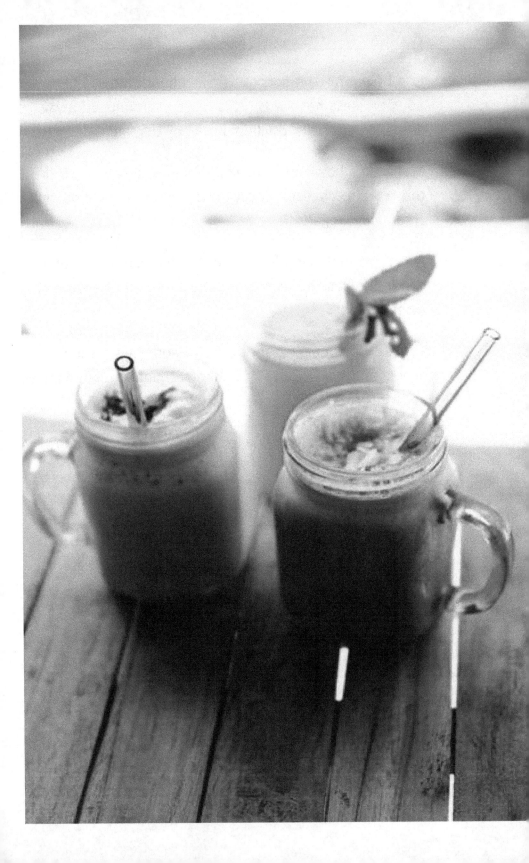

Banana-Strawberry Smoothie

6 Servings

Preparation Time: 5 minutes

Ingredients

- 6 Bananas, sliced
- 6 cups Kale
- 6 cups Plant-based milk
- 6 cups Strawberries

Directions and

- In a blender, add bananas, strawberries, kale, and milk and blend until smooth.

- Divide between glasses and serve.

Simple Pear Oatmeal

4 Servings

Preparation Time: 20 minutes

Ingredients

- 1 ¼ cups Apple cider
- ⅔ cup Rolled oats
- 1 tsp ground Cinnamon
- 1 tbsp pure Date syrup
- 1 Pear, peeled, cored, and chopped

Directions

- Add the apple cider into a pot over medium heat and bring to a boil.

- Add in the pear, oats, and cinnamon. Lower the heat and simmer for 3-4 minutes until the oatmeal thickens.

- Divide between bowls and drizzle with date syrup. Serve immediately.

Cranberry Oat Cookies

4 Servings

Preparation Time: 20 minutes

Ingredients

- ½ cup Rolled oats
- 2 tbsps Pure date sugar
- ¼ cup Applesauce
- 2 tbsps Dried cranberries
- 1 tbsp Whole-wheat flour
- ½ tsp Baking powder

Directions

- Mix the oats, flour, baking powder, and sugar in a bowl.

- Add in applesauce and cranberries. Stir until well combined.

- Make 4 cookies out of the mixture and microwave for 1 ½ minutes. Allow cooling before serving.

Matcha Smoothie

6 Servings

Preparation Time: 5 minutes

Ingredients

- 1 cup chopped Pineapple
- 1 cup chopped spinach
- ½ avocado
- ½ cup Almond milk
- 1 tsp Matcha green tea powder
- 1 cup chopped mango

Directions

- Put everything in a blender until smooth, adding 1 cup water if needed.

- In a blender, place the pineapple, mango, spinach, avocado, almond milk, water, and matcha powder. Blend until smooth.

- Divide between 6 glasses and serve.

DRINKS

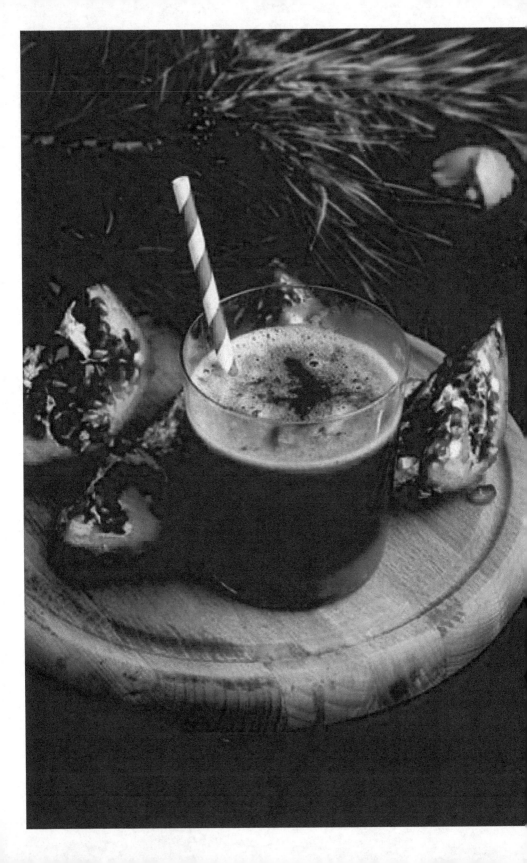

Energizing Cinnamon Detox Tonic

2 Servings

Preparation Time: 30 minutes

Ingredients

- 4 sticks of cinnamon 2 inches each
- 1 small lemon slice
- 1/8 teaspoon of cayenne pepper
- 1/8 teaspoon of ground turmeric
- 1 teaspoon of maple syrup
- 1 teaspoon of apple cider vinegar
- 2 cups of boiling water

Directions

- Pour the boiling water into a small saucepan, add and stir the cinnamon sticks, then let it rest for 8 to 10 minutes before covering the pan.
- Pass the mixture through a strainer and into the liquid; add the cayenne pepper, turmeric, cinnamon and stir properly.
- Add the maple syrup, vinegar, and lemon slice.
- Add and stir an infused lemon and serve immediately.

Warm Pomegranate Punch

10 Servings

Preparation Time: 35 minutes

Ingredients

- 3 cinnamon sticks, each about 3 inches long
- 12 whole cloves
- 1/2 cup of coconut sugar
- 1/3 cup of lemon juice
- 32 fluid ounce of pomegranate juice
- 32 fluid ounce of apple juice, unsweetened
- 16 fluid ounce of brewed tea

Directions

- Using a 4-quart slow cooker, pour the lemon juice, pomegranate juice, apple juice, tea, and then sugar.
- Wrap the whole cloves and cinnamon stick in cheesecloth, tie its corners with a string, and immerse it in the liquid present in the slow cooker.
- Then cover it with the lid, plug in the slow cooker and let it cook at the low heat setting for 3 hours or until it is heated thoroughly.
- When done, discard the cheesecloth bag and serve it hot or cold.

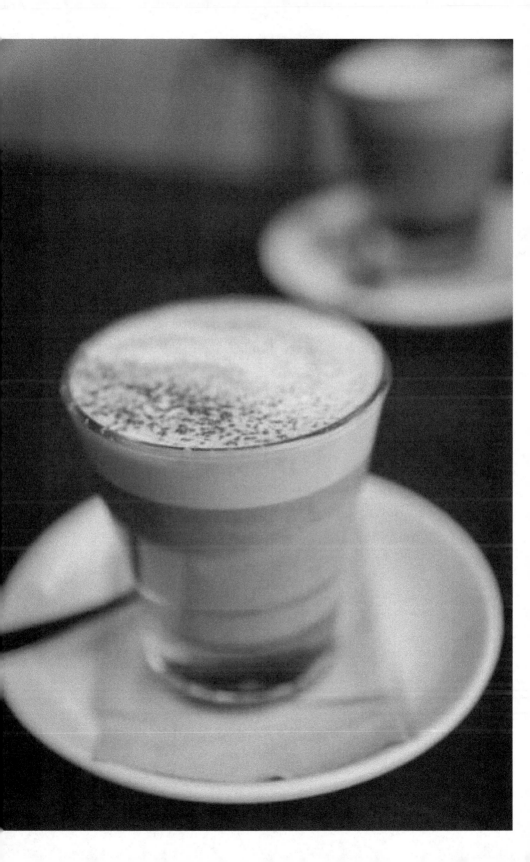

Rich Truffle Hot Chocolate

4 Servings

Preparation Time: 35 minutes

Ingredients

- 1/3 cup of cocoa powder, unsweetened
- 1/3 cup of coconut sugar
- 1/8 teaspoon of salt
- 1/8 teaspoon of ground cinnamon
- 1 teaspoon of vanilla extract, unsweetened
- 32 fluid ounce of coconut milk

Directions

- Using a 2 quarts slow cooker, add all the ingredients, and stir properly.
- Cover it with the lid, then plug in the slow cooker and cook it for 2 hours on the high heat setting or until it is heated thoroughly.
- When done, serve right away.

Warm Spiced Lemon Drink

12 Servings

Preparation Time: 30 minutes

Ingredients

- 1 cinnamon stick, about 3 inches long
- 1/2 teaspoon of whole cloves
- 2 cups of coconut sugar
- 4 fluid of ounce pineapple juice
- 1/2 cup and 2 tablespoons of lemon juice
- 12 fluid ounce of orange juice
- 2 1/2 quarts of water

Directions

- Pour water into a 6-quarts slow cooker and stir the sugar and lemon juice properly.
- Wrap the cinnamon, the whole cloves in cheesecloth, and tie its corners with string.
- Immerse this cheesecloth bag in the liquid present in the slow cooker and cover it with the lid.
- Then plug in the slow cooker and let it cook on a high heat setting for 2 hours or until it is heated thoroughly.
- When done, discard the cheesecloth bag and serve the drink hot or cold.

Pumpkin Spice Frappuccino

2 Servings

Preparation Time: 5 minutes

Ingredients

- ½ teaspoon ground ginger
- 1/8 teaspoon allspice
- ½ teaspoon ground cinnamon
- 2 tablespoons coconut sugar
- 1/8 teaspoon nutmeg
- ¼ teaspoon ground cloves
- 1 teaspoon vanilla extract, unsweetened
- 2 teaspoons instant coffee
- 2 cups almond milk, unsweetened
- 1 cup of ice cubes

Directions

- Place all the ingredients in the order in a food processor or blender and then pulse for 2 to 3 minutes at high speed until smooth.
- Pour the Frappuccino into two glasses and then serve.

Cookie Dough Milkshake

2 Servings

Preparation Time: 5 minutes

Ingredients

- 2 tablespoons cookie dough
- 5 dates, pitted
- 2 teaspoons chocolate chips
- 1/2 teaspoon vanilla extract, unsweetened
- 1/2 cup almond milk, unsweetened
- 1 ½ cups almond milk ice cubes

Directions

- Place all the ingredients in the order in a food processor or blender and then pulse for 2 to 3 minutes at high speed until smooth.
- Pour the milkshake into two glasses and then serve with some cookie dough balls.

LUNCH

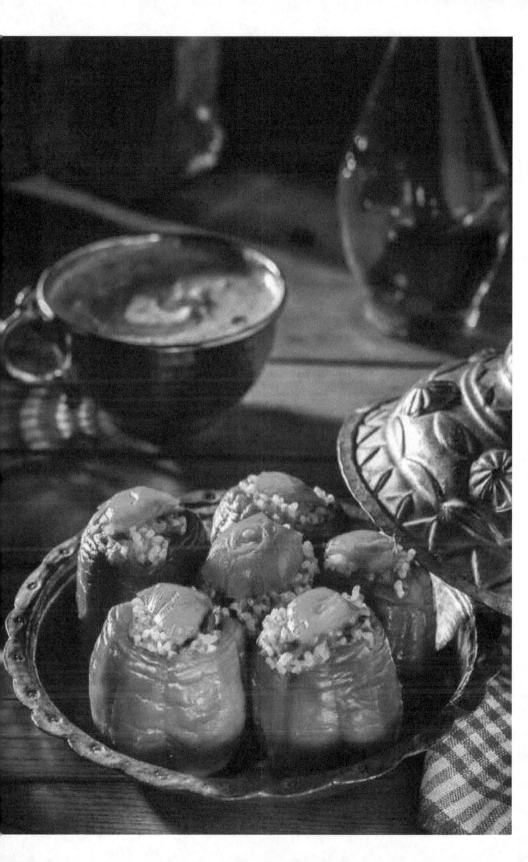

Mushroom & Green Bean Biryani

6 Servings

Preparation Time: 50 minutes

Ingredients

- 1 cup Brown rice
- 3 tbsps Plant butter
- 3 medium white onions, chopped
- 6 Garlic cloves, minced
- 1 tsp Ginger puree
- 1 tbsp Turmeric powder + for dusting
- ¼ tsp Cinnamon powder
- 2 tsps Gram masala
- ½ tsp Cardamom powder
- ½ tsp Cayenne powder
- ½ tsp Cumin powder
- 1 tsp Smoked paprika
- 3 large Tomatoes, diced
- 1 tbsp Tomato puree
- 1 cup chopped Cremini mushrooms
- 1 cup chopped Mustard greens
- 1 cup Plant-based yogurt
- 2 green Chilies, minced

Directions

- Melt the butter in a large pot and sauté the onions until softened, 2 minutes.

- Mix in the garlic, ginger, turmeric, cardamom powder, gram masala, cardamom powder, cayenne pepper, cumin powder, paprika, and salt. Stir-fry for 1-2 minutes.

- Stir in the tomatoes, green chili, tomato puree, and mushrooms. Once boiling, mix in the rice and cover it with water.

- Cover the pot and cook over medium heat until the liquid absorbs and the rice is tender for 15-20 minutes.

- Open the lid and fluff in the mustard greens and half of the parsley. Dish the food, top with the coconut yogurt, garnish with the remaining parsley, and serve warm.

Kale & Mushroom Pierogis

6 Servings

Preparation Time: 45 minutes

Ingredients

Stuffing

- 2 tbsps plant butter
- 2 garlic cloves, finely chopped
- 1 small red onion, finely chopped
- 3 oz baby Bella mushrooms, sliced
- 2 oz fresh kale
- ½ tsp salt
- ¼ tsp freshly ground black pepper
- ½ cup dairy-free cream cheese
- 2 oz plant-based Parmesan, grated

Pierogi

- 1 tbsp flax seed powder
- ½ cup almond flour
- 4 tbsps coconut flour
- ½ tsp salt
- 1 tsp baking powder
- 1 ½ cups grated plant-based Parmesan
- 5 tbsps plant butter
- Olive oil for brushing

Directions

- Add the plant butter into a pan and melt over medium heat, then add and sauté the garlic, red onion, mushrooms, and kale until the mushrooms brown.

- Season the mixture with salt and black pepper and reduce the heat to low.

- Mix in the cream cheese and plant-based Parmesan cheese and simmer for 1 minute.

- Turn the heat off and set the filling aside to cool.

- Make the pierogis: In a small bowl, mix the flax seed powder with 3 tbsps water and allow sitting for 5 minutes.

- In a bowl, combine almond flour, coconut flour, salt, and baking powder.

- Put a small pan over low heat, add, and melt the plant-based Parmesan cheese and plant butter while stirring continuously until smooth batter forms. Turn the heat off.

- Pour the vegan "flax egg" into the cream mixture, continue stirring while adding the flour mixture until a firm dough forms. Mold the dough into four balls, place on a chopping board, and use a rolling pin to flatten each into ½ inch thin round pieces.

- Spread a generous amount of stuffing on one-half of each dough, then fold over the filling, and seal the dough with your fingers. Brush with olive oil, place on a baking sheet, and bake for 20 minutes at 380 F. Serve with salad.

Vegan Mushroom Pizza

6 Servings

Preparation Time: 35 minutes

Ingredients

- 2 tsps Plant butter
- 1 cup Tomato sauce
- 1 cup plant-based Parmesan cheese
- 5-6 Basil leaves
- 1 cup chopped button Mushrooms
- ½ cup sliced mixed Bell peppers
- Salt and Black pepper to taste
- 1 pizza crust

Directions

- Melt plant butter in a pan and sauté mushrooms and bell peppers for 10 minutes until softened.

- Season with salt and black pepper.

- Put the pizza crust on a pizza pan, spread the tomato sauce all over, and scatter vegetables evenly on top.

- Spread with plant-based Parmesan cheese. Bake for 20 minutes until the cheese has melted.

- Garnish with basil and serve.

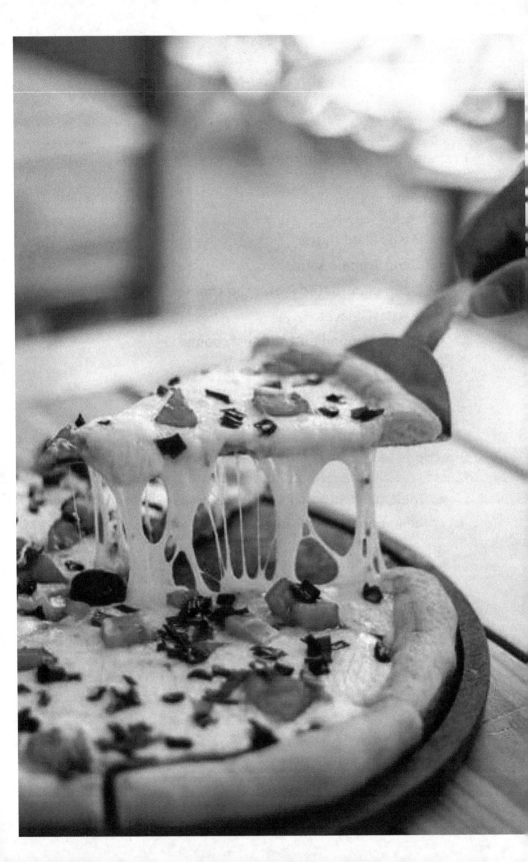

Grilled Zucchini with Spinach Avocado Pesto

6 Servings

Preparation Time: 20 minutes

Ingredients

- 3 oz spinach, chopped
- ¾ cup olive oil
- 2 zucchinis, sliced
- 1 tbsp fresh lemon juice
- 2 tbsps melted plant butter
- 1 ½ lbs tempeh slices
- 1 ripe avocado, chopped
- Juice of 1 lemon
- 1 garlic clove, minced
- 2 oz pecans
- Salt and black pepper to taste

Directions

- Put the spinach in a blender along with the avocado, lemon juice, garlic, and pecans.

- Blend until smooth and then season with salt and black pepper.

- Put the olive oil and process a little more. Pour the pesto into a bowl and set aside.

- Place zucchini in a bowl. Season with the remaining lemon juice, salt, black pepper, and the plant butter.

- Also, season the tempeh with salt and black pepper, and brush with olive oil.

- Preheat a grill pan and cook both the tempeh and zucchini slices until browned on both sides.

- Plate the tempeh and zucchini, spoon some pesto to the side, and serve immediately.

Eggplant Fries with Chili Aioli & Beet Salad

6 Servings

Preparation Time: 35 minutes

Ingredients

Eggplant Fries

- 2 tbsps flax seed powder

- 2 eggplants, sliced
- 2 cups almond flour
- Salt and black pepper to taste
- 2 tbsps olive oil

Spicy Aioli

- 1 tbsp flax seed powder

- 2 garlic cloves, minced
- ¾ cup light olive oil
- ½ tsp red chili flakes
- 1 tbsp freshly squeezed lemon juice
- 3 tbsps dairy-free yogurt

Beet salad

- 3½ oz beets, peeled and thinly cut

- 3½ oz red cabbage, grated
- 2 tbsps fresh cilantro
- 2 tbsps olive oil
- 1 tbsp freshly squeezed lime juice
- Salt and black pepper to taste

Directions

- Preheat oven to 400 F.

- In a bowl, combine the flax seed powder with 6 tbsps water and allow sitting to thicken for 5 minutes.

- In a deep plate, mix almond flour, salt, and black pepper. Dip the eggplant slices into the vegan "flax egg," then in the almond flour, and then in the vegan "flax egg," and finally in the flour mixture.

- Place the eggplants on a greased baking sheet and drizzle with olive oil. Bake until the fries are crispy and brown, about 15 minutes.

- For the aioli, mix the flax seed powder with 3 tbsps water in a bowl and set aside to thicken for 5 minutes. Whisk in garlic while pouring in the olive oil gradually.

- Stir in red chili flakes, salt, black pepper, lemon juice, and dairy-free yogurt.

- Adjust the taste with salt, garlic, or yogurt as desired.

- For the beet salad, in a salad bowl, combine the beets, red cabbage, cilantro, olive oil, lime juice, salt, and black pepper.

- Use two spoons to toss the ingredients until properly combined.

- Serve the eggplant fries with the chili aioli and beet salad.

Tofu Skewers with Salsa Verde & Squash Mash

6 Servings

Preparation Time: 20 minutes

Ingredients

- 7 tbsps fresh Cilantro, finely chopped
- 1 tbsp melted plant butter
- 3 cups butternut squash, cubed
- ½ cup cold plant butter
- 2 oz grated plant-based Parmesan
- 4 tbsps fresh Basil, finely chopped
- 2 Garlic cloves
- Juice of ½ Lemon
- 4 tbsps Capers
- 2/3 cup Olive oil
- 1 lb extra firm tofu, cubed
- ½ tbsp sugar-free BBQ sauce

Directions

- Add cilantro, basil, garlic, lemon juice, capers, olive oil, salt, and pepper in a blender.

- Process until smooth; set aside. Thread the tofu cubes on wooden skewers.

- Season with salt and brush with BBQ sauce.

- Melt plant butter in a grill pan and fry the tofu until browned. Remove to a plate.

- Pour the squash into a pot, add some lightly salted water, and bring the vegetable to a boil until soft, about 6 minutes.

- Drain and pour into a bowl. Add the cold plant butter, plant-based Parmesan cheese, salt, and black pepper.

- Mash the vegetable with an immersion blender until the consistency of mashed potatoes is achieved.

- Serve the tofu skewers with the mashed cauliflower and salsa Verde.

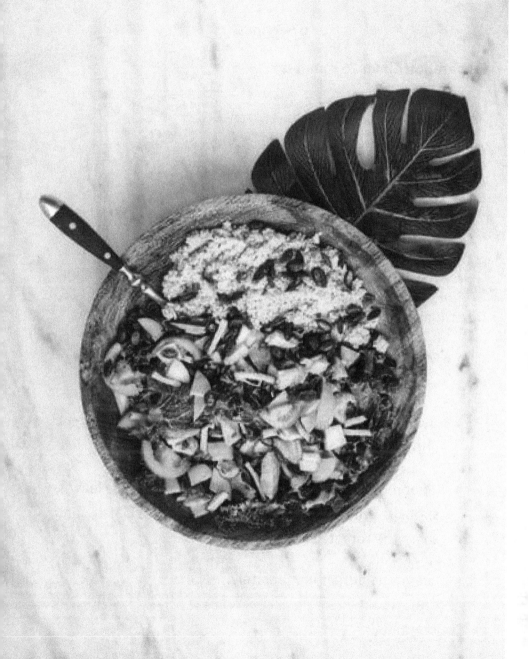

Mushroom Lettuce Wraps

6 Servings

Preparation Time: 25 minutes

Ingredients

- 2 tbsps Plant butter
- 1 iceberg Lettuce, leaves extracted
- 1 cup grated plant-based cheddar
- 1 large Tomato, sliced
- 4 oz baby Bella mushrooms, sliced
- 1 ½ lbs Tofu, crumbled

Directions

- Melt the plant butter in a pan, add in mushrooms and sauté until browned and tender, about 6 minutes.

- Transfer to a plate. Add the tofu to the pan and cook until brown, about 10 minutes.

- Spoon the tofu and mushrooms into the lettuce leaves, sprinkle with the plant-based cheddar cheese, and share the tomato slices on top.

- Serve the burger immediately.

Chili Bean & Brown Rice Tortillas

6 Servings

Preparation Time: 50 minutes

Ingredients

- 1 cup Brown rice
- 4 whole-wheat flour tortillas, warmed
- 1 cup Salsa
- 1 cup Coconut cream for topping
- 1 cup grated plant-based cheddar
- Salt and Black pepper to taste
- 1 tbsp Olive oil
- 1 medium red Onion, chopped
- 1 green bell Pepper, diced
- 2 Garlic cloves, minced
- 1 tbsp Chili powder
- 1 tsp Cumin powder
- 1/8 tsp red Chili flakes
- 1 (15 oz) can Black beans, rinsed

Directions

- Add 2 cups of water and brown rice to a medium pot, season with some salt, and cook over medium heat until the water absorbs and the rice is tender, 15 to 20 minutes.

- Heat the olive oil in a medium skillet over medium heat and sauté the onion, bell pepper, and garlic until softened and fragrant, 3 minutes.

- Mix in the chili powder, cumin powder, red chili flakes, and season with salt and black pepper.

- Cook for 1 minute or until the food releases fragrance. Stir in the brown rice, black beans, and allow warming through, 3 minutes. Lay the tortillas on a clean, flat surface and divide the rice mixture in the center of each.

- Top with the salsa, coconut cream, and plant cheddar cheese. Fold the sides and ends of the tortillas over the filling to secure. Serve immediately.

SNACKS & SIDES

Mashed Broccoli with Roasted Garlic

8 Servings

Preparation time: 45 minutes

Ingredients

- 1 head garlic
- 4 tbsps olive oil + for garnish
- 2 head broccoli, cut into florets
- 2 tsps salt
- 8 oz plant butter
- ½ tsp dried thyme
- Juice and zest of half a lemon
- 8 tbsps coconut cream

Directions

- Preheat oven to 400 F.

- Use a knife to cut a ¼ inch off the top of the garlic cloves, drizzle with olive oil, and wrap in aluminum foil.

- Place on a baking sheet and roast for 30 minutes. Remove and set aside when ready.

- Pour the broccoli into a pot, add 3 cups of water, and 1 teaspoon of salt. Bring to a boil until tender, about 7 minutes.

- Drain and transfer the broccoli to a bowl. Add the plant butter, thyme, lemon juice and zest, coconut cream, and olive oil.

- Use an immersion blender to puree the ingredients until smooth and nice.

- Spoon the mash into serving bowls and garnish with some olive oil. Serve.

Spicy Pistachio Dip

8 Servings

Preparation time: 10 minutes

Ingredients

- 6 oz toasted pistachios + for garnish
- 6 tbsps coconut cream
- ½ cup water
- Juice of half a lemon
- 1 tsp smoked paprika
- Cayenne pepper to taste
- 1 tsp salt
- 1 cup olive oil

Directions

- Pour the pistachios, coconut cream, water, lemon juice, paprika, cayenne pepper, and salt.

- Puree the ingredients at high speed until smooth.

- Add the olive oil and puree a little further. Manage the consistency of the dip by adding more oil or water.

- Spoon the dip into little bowls, garnish with some pistachios, and serve with julienned celery and carrots.

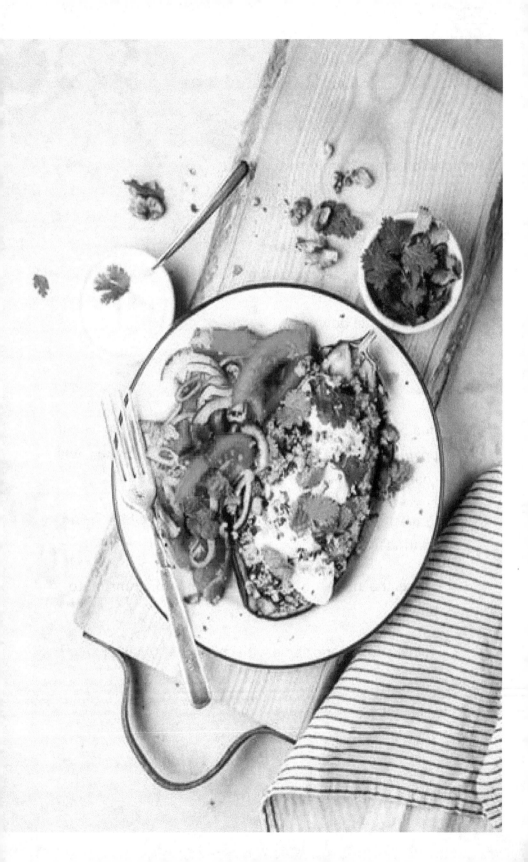

Paprika Roasted Nuts

8 Servings

Preparation time: 10 minutes

Ingredients

- 16 oz walnuts and pecans
- 2 tsps salt
- 2 tbsps coconut oil
- 2 tsps cumin powder
- 2 tsps paprika powder

Directions

- In a bowl, mix walnuts, pecans, salt, coconut oil, cumin powder, and paprika powder until the nuts are well coated with spice and oil.

- Pour the mixture into a pan and toast while stirring continually.

- Once the nuts are fragrant and brown, transfer to a bowl.

- Allow cooling and serve with chilled berry juice.

Mixed Vegetables with Basil

8 Servings

Preparation time: 40 minutes

Ingredients

- 4 medium zucchinis, chopped
- 4 medium yellow squash, chopped
- 2 red onions, cut into 1-inch wedges
- 2 red bell peppers, diced
- 2 cups cherry tomatoes, halved
- 8 tbsps olive oil
- Salt and black pepper to taste
- 6 garlic cloves, minced
- 1 ½ cups whole-wheat breadcrumbs
- 2 lemons, zested
- ½ cup chopped fresh basil

Directions

- Preheat the oven to 450 F.

- Lightly grease a large baking sheet with cooking spray.

- In a medium bowl, add the zucchini, yellow squash, red onion, bell pepper, tomatoes, olive oil, salt, black pepper, and garlic.

- Toss well and spread the mixture on the baking sheet.

- Roast in the oven for 25 to 30 minutes or until the vegetables are tender while stirring every 5 minutes.

- Meanwhile, heat the olive oil in a medium skillet and sauté the garlic until fragrant. Mix in the breadcrumbs, lemon zest, and basil. Cook for 2 to 3 minutes.

- Remove the vegetables from the oven and toss in the breadcrumb's mixture. Serve.

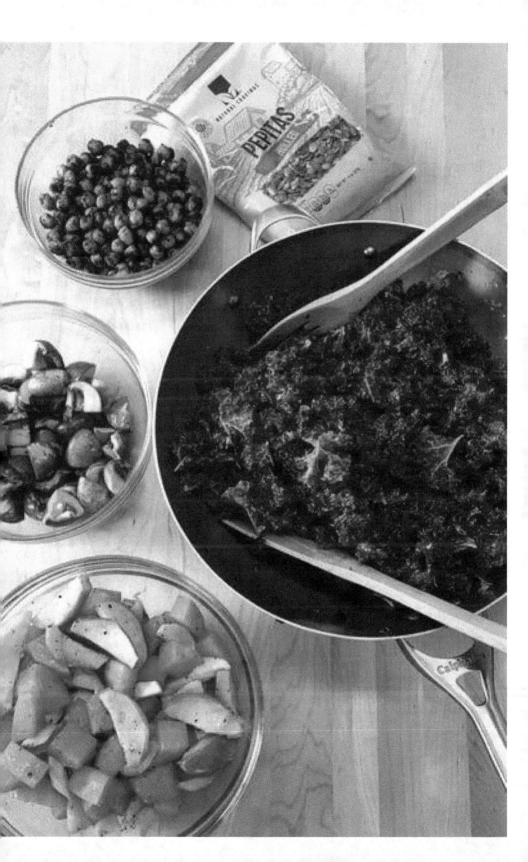

Onion Rings & Kale Dip

8 Servings

Preparation time: 25 minutes

Ingredients

- 2 onions, sliced into rings
- 2 tbsps flaxseed meal + 3 tbsps water
- 2 cups almond flour
- 1 cup grated plant-based Parmesan
- 4 tsps garlic powder
- 1 tbsp sweet paprika powder
- 4 oz chopped kale
- 4 tbsps olive oil
- 4 tbsps dried cilantro
- 2 tbsps dried oregano
- Salt and black pepper to taste
- 2 cups tofu mayonnaise
- 8 tbsps coconut cream
- Juice of a lemon

Directions

- Preheat oven to 400 F.

- In a bowl, mix the flaxseed meal and water and leave the mixture to thicken and fully absorb for 5 minutes.

- In another bowl, combine almond flour, plant-based Parmesan cheese, half of the garlic powder, sweet paprika, and salt.

- Line a baking sheet with parchment paper in readiness for the rings.

- When the vegan "flax egg" is ready, dip in the onion rings one after another, and then into the almond flour mixture.

- Place the rings on the baking sheet and grease them with cooking spray.

- Bake for 15-20 minutes or until golden brown and crispy.

- Remove the onion rings into a serving bowl.

- Put kale in a food processor.

- Add in olive oil, cilantro, oregano, remaining garlic powder, salt, black pepper, tofu mayonnaise, coconut cream, and lemon juice; puree until nice and smooth

- . Allow the dip to sit for about 10 minutes for the flavors to develop. After, serve the dip with the crispy onion rings.

Sesame Cabbage Sauté

4 Servings

Preparation time: 15 minutes

Ingredients

- 2 tbsps soy sauce
- 1 tbsp toasted sesame oil
- 1 tbsp hot sauce
- ½ tbsp pure date sugar
- ½ tbsp olive oil
- 1 head green cabbage, shredded
- 2 carrots, julienned
- 3 green onions, thinly sliced
- 2 garlic cloves, minced
- 1 tbsp fresh grated ginger
- Salt and black pepper to taste
- 1 tbsp sesame seeds

Directions a

- In a small bowl, mix the soy sauce, sesame oil, hot sauce, and date sugar.
- Heat the olive oil in a large skillet and sauté the cabbage, carrots, green onion, garlic, and ginger until softened, 5 minutes.
- Mix in the prepared sauce and toss well. Cook for 1 to 2 minutes.
- Dish the food and garnish with the sesame seeds.

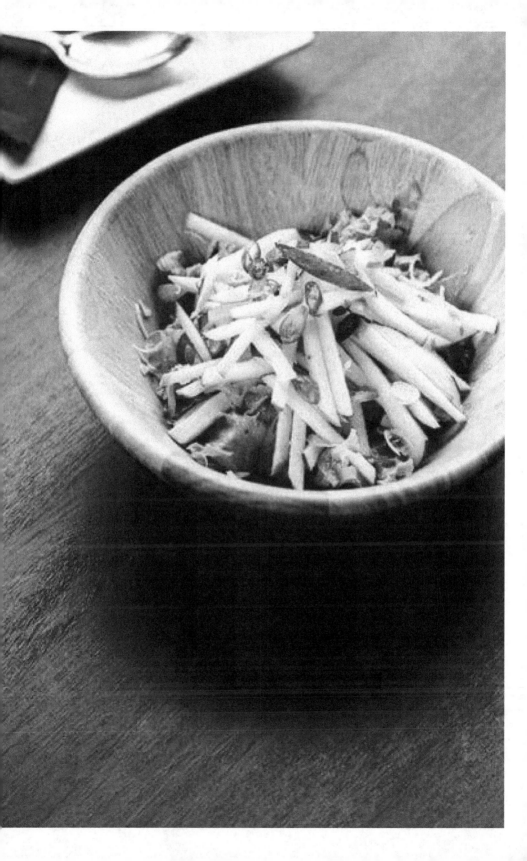

Tomatoes Stuffed with Chickpeas & Quinoa

4 Servings

Preparation time: 50 minutes

Ingredients

- 8 medium tomatoes
- ¾ cup quinoa, rinsed and drained
- 1 ½ cups water
- 1 tbsp olive oil
- 1 small onion, diced
- 3 garlic cloves, minced
- 1 cup chopped spinach
- 1 (7 oz) can chickpeas, drained
- ½ cup chopped fresh basil

Directions

- Preheat the oven to 400 F.

- Cut off the heads of tomatoes and use a paring knife to scoop the inner pulp of the tomatoes.

- Season with some olive oil, salt, and black pepper.

- Add the quinoa and water to a medium pot, season with salt, and cook until the quinoa is tender and the water absorbs for 10 to 15 minutes.

- Fluff and set aside.

- Heat the remaining olive oil in a skillet and sauté the onion and garlic for 30 seconds. Mix in the spinach and cook until wilted, 2 minutes.

- Stir in the basil, chickpeas, and quinoa; allow warming from 2 minutes.

- Spoon the mixture into the tomatoes, place the tomatoes into the baking dish and bake in the oven for 20 minutes or until the tomatoes soften.

- Remove the tomatoes from the oven and dish the food.

SOUPS & SALADS

Broccoli Fennel Soup

6 Servings

Preparation Time: 25 minutes

Ingredients

- 1 Fennel bulb, chopped
- 1 Garlic clove
- 1 cup Cashew cream cheese
- 3 oz Plant butter
- ½ cup chopped Fresh oregano
- 10 oz Broccoli, cut into florets
- 3 cups Vegetable stock
- Salt and Black pepper to taste

Directions

- Put the fennel and broccoli into a pot, and cover with the vegetable stock.

- Bring the ingredients to a boil over medium heat until the vegetables are soft, about 10 minutes.

- Season the liquid with salt and black pepper, and drop in the garlic. Simmer the soup for 5 to 7 minutes and turn the heat off.

- Put the cream cheese, plant butter, and oregano into the soup; puree the ingredients with an immersion blender until completely smooth.

- Adjust the taste with salt and black pepper. Spoon the soup into serving bowls and serve.

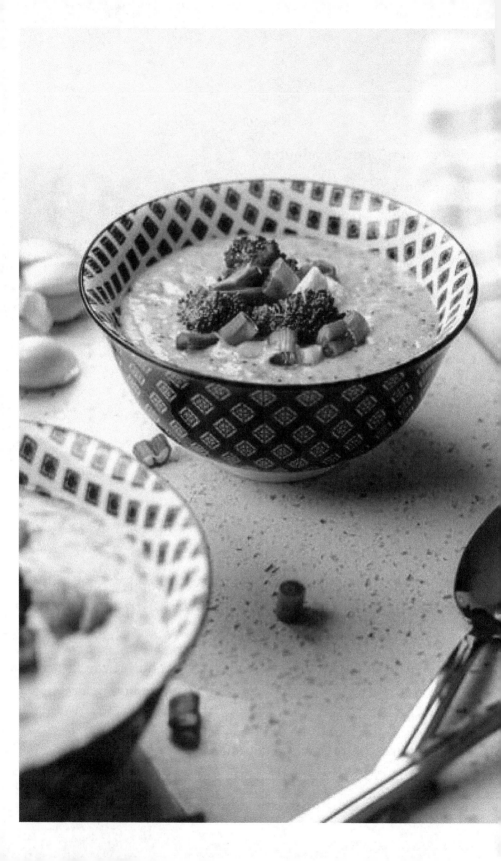

Asian-Style Bean Soup

6 Servings

Preparation Time: 55 minutes

Ingredients

- 1 cup canned Cannellini beans
- 2 cubed Sweet potatoes
- 1 cup sliced zucchini
- Salt and Black pepper to taste
- 4 cups Vegetable stock
- 1 bunch Spinach, chopped
- Toasted Sesame seeds
- 2 tsps Curry powder
- 2 tsps Olive oil
- 1 red Onion, diced
- 1 tbsp Minced fresh ginger

Directions

- Mix the beans with 1 tsp of curry powder until well combined.

- Heat the oil in a pot over medium heat.

- Put the onion and ginger and cook for 5 minutes until soft.

- Add in sweet potatoes and cook for 10 minutes. Put in zucchini and cook for 5 minutes.

- Season with the remaining curry, pepper, and salt.

- Pour in the stock and bring to a boil. Lower the heat and simmer for 25 minutes.

- Stir in beans and spinach. Cook until the spinach wilts and remove from the heat.

- Garnish with sesame seeds to serve.

Spicy Bean Soup

6 Servings

Preparation Time: 40 minutes

Ingredients

- 2 tbsps Olive oil
- 1 (15.5-oz) can Cannellini beans, drained
- 5 cups vegetable broth
- ¼ tsp crushed Red pepper
- Salt and Black pepper to taste
- 3 cups chopped baby spinach
- 1 medium Onion, chopped
- 2 large Garlic cloves, minced
- 1 Carrot, chopped

Directions

- Warm the oil in a pot over medium heat.

- Place in carrot, onion, and garlic and cook for 3 minutes. Put in beans, broth, red pepper, salt, and black pepper and stir.

- Bring to a boil, then lower the heat and simmer for 25 minutes.

- Stir in baby spinach and cook for 5 minutes until the spinach wilts. Serve warm.

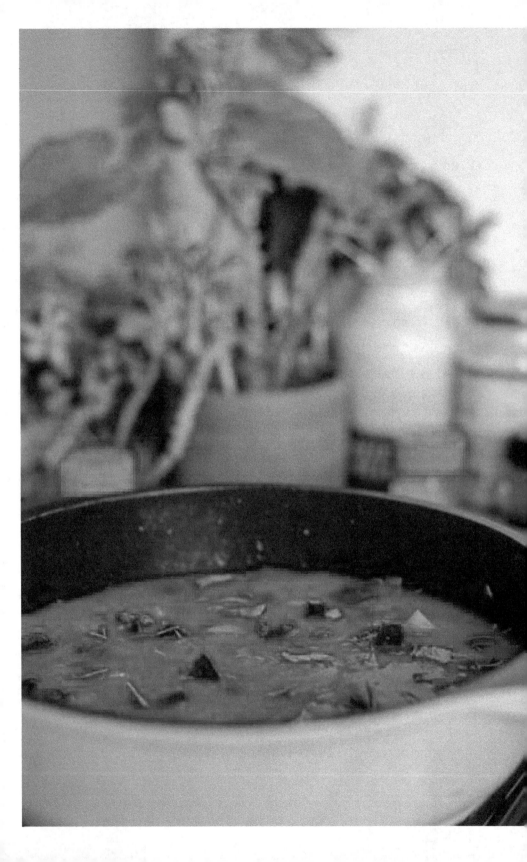

Rice Wine Mushroom Soup

6 Servings

Preparation Time: 25 minutes

Ingredients

- 2 tbsps Olive oil
- 3 tbsps Rice wine
- 2 tbsps Soy sauce
- 4 cups vegetable broth
- Salt and Black pepper to taste
- 2 tbsps parsley, chopped
- 4 green onions, chopped
- 1 Carrot, chopped
- 8 oz Shiitake mushrooms, sliced

Directions

- Warm the oil in a pot over medium heat.

- Add the green onions and carrot and cook for 5 minutes.

- Stir in mushrooms, rice wine, soy sauce, broth, salt, and pepper.

- Bring to a boil, then lower the heat and simmer for 15 minutes. Top with parsley and serve warm.

Minty Eggplant Salad

6 Servings

Preparation time: 45 minutes

Ingredients

- 1 Lemon, half zested and juiced, half cut into wedges
- ¼ tsp Ground nutmeg
- Sea salt to taste
- 2 tbsps Capers
- 1 tbsp chopped Green olives
- 1 Garlic clove, pressed
- 2 tbsps fresh Mint, finely chopped
- 2 cups Watercress, chopped
- 1 tsp Olive oil
- 1Eeggplant, chopped
- ½ tsp Ground cumin
- ½ tsp Ground ginger
- ¼ tsp Turmeric

Directions

- In a pan over medium heat, warm the oil.

- Place the eggplant and cook for 5 minutes.

- Put in cumin, ginger, turmeric, nutmeg, and salt. Cook for another 10 minutes.

- Stir in lemon zest, lemon juice, capers, olives, garlic, and mint. Cook for 1-2 minutes more.

- Place some watercress on each plate and top with the eggplant mixture. Serve it.

Potato & Green Bean Salad

4 Servings

Preparation time: 30 minutes

Ingredients

- 1 ½ lbs small Potatoes, unpeeled
- 2 tbsps Soy sauce
- 1 tbsp Rice vinegar
- ¾ cup Coconut milk
- 3 tbsps chopped roasted peanuts
- 1 cup frozen Green beans, thawed
- ½ cup shredded Carrots
- 4 green onions, chopped
- 1 tbsp Grapeseed oil
- 1 Garlic clove, minced
- 1/3 cup Peanut butter
- ½ tsp Asian chili paste

Directions

- Put the potatoes in a pot with a boil in salted water and cook for 20 minutes. Drain and let cool.

- Chop the potatoes into chunks and place them in a bowl.

- Stir in green beans, carrots, and green onions. Set aside.

- Heat oil in a pot over medium heat.

- Place in garlic and cook for 30 seconds.

- Add in peanut butter, chili, soy sauce, vinegar, coconut milk. Cook for 5 minutes, stirring often.

- Pour over the potatoes and toss to coat. Serve garnished with peanuts.

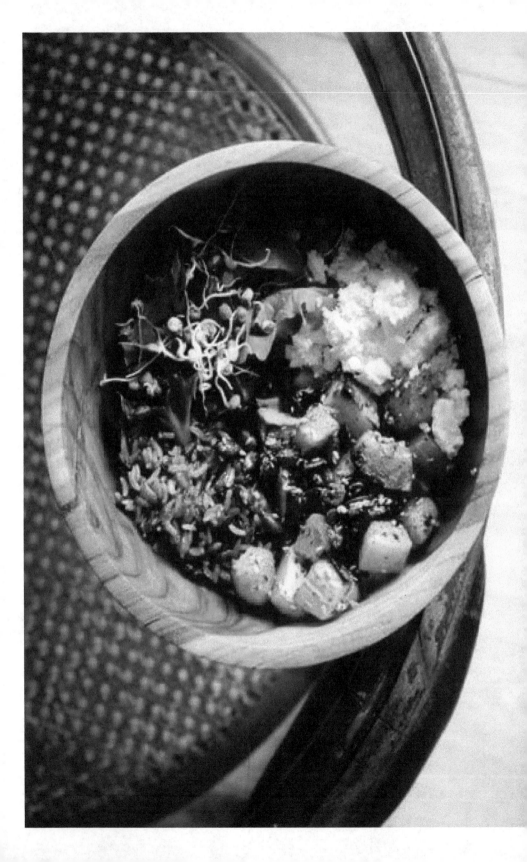

Artichoke & Potato Salad

6 Servings

Preparation time: 30 minutes

Ingredients

- 1 (10-oz) package frozen Artichoke hearts, cooked
- 1 ½ lbs Potatoes, chopped
- 2 cups halved cherry tomatoes
- ½ cup sweet corn
- 3 Green onions, minced
- 1 tbsp minced fresh parsley
- ⅓ cup Olive oil
- 2 tbsps fresh Lemon juice
- 1 Garlic clove, minced
- Salt and Black pepper to taste

Directions

- Put the potatoes in a pot with salted water and boil for 15 minutes. Drain and remove to a bowl.
- Cut the artichokes by quarts and mix them into the potato bowl.
- Stir in tomatoes, corn, green onions, and parsley. Set aside.
- Whisk the oil, lemon juice, garlic, salt, and pepper in a bowl.
- Pour over the potatoes and toss to coat. Let sit for 20 minutes. And serve.

Colorful Quinoa Salad

6 Servings

Preparation Time: 15 minutes

Ingredients

- 1 cup Canned mandarin oranges in juice, drained
- 2 cups Cooked tricolor quinoa
- 1 cup Diced yellow summer squash
- 1 Red bell pepper, diced
- ½ Red onion, sliced
- ½ cup Dried cranberries
- ½ cup Slivered almonds
- 3 tbsps Olive oil
- Juice of 1 ½ lemons
- 1 tsp Garlic powder
- ½ tsp Dried oregano
- 1 bunch baby spinach

Directions

- Mix the oil, lemon juice, garlic powder, and oregano in a bowl.
- In another bowl, place the spinach and pour over the dressing, toss to coat.
- Stir in quinoa, oranges, squash, bell pepper, and red onion.
- Share into bowls and garnish with cranberries and almonds to serve.

DINNER

Traditional Cilantro Pilaf

6 Servings

Preparation Time: 30 minutes

Ingredients

- 3 tbsps Olive oil
- 1 ½ tsps ground Fennel seeds
- ½ tsp ground Cumin
- Salt and black pepper to taste
- 3 tbsps minced fresh cilantro
- 1 onion, minced
- 1 carrot, chopped
- 2 garlic cloves, minced
- 1 cup wild rice

Directions

- Heat the oil in a pot over medium heat. Place in onion, carrot, and garlic and sauté for 5 minutes. Stir in rice, fennel seeds, cumin, and 2 cups water.

- Bring to a boil, then lower the heat and simmer for 20 minutes.

- Remove to a bowl and fluff using a fork.

- Serve topped with cilantro and black pepper.

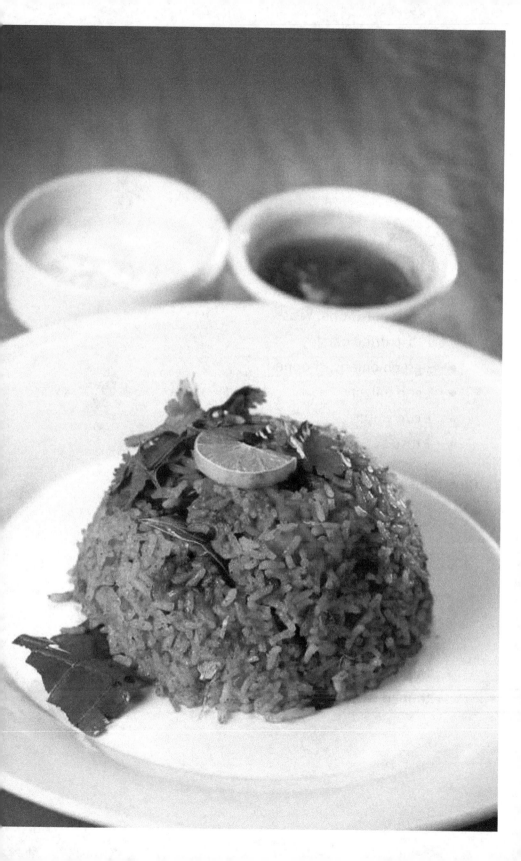

Oriental Bulgur & White Beans

6 Servings

Preparation Time: 55 minutes

Ingredients

- 2 tbsps Olive oil
- Salt to taste
- 1 ½ cups cooked white Beans
- 1 tbsp nutritional Yeast
- 1 tbsp dried parsley
- 3 green onions, chopped
- 1 cup bulgur
- 1 cup water
- 1 tbsp Soy sauce

Directions

- Heat the oil in a pot over medium heat.

- Place in green onions and sauté for 3 minutes.

- Stir in bulgur, water, soy sauce, and salt. Bring to a boil, then lower the heat and simmer for 20-22 minutes.

- Mix in beans and yeast. Cook for 5 minutes. Serve topped with parsley.

Celery Buckwheat Croquettes

6 Servings

Preparation Time: 25 minutes

Ingredients

- ¾ cup cooked Buckwheat groats
- 1 celery Stalk, chopped
- ¼ cup shredded Carrots
- 1/3 cup whole-wheat flour
- ¼ cup chopped fresh parsley
- Salt and black pepper to taste
- ½ cup cooked brown rice
- 3 tbsps olive oil
- ¼ cup minced onion

Directions

- Mix the groats and rice in a bowl. Set aside. Heat 1 tbsp of oil in a pan over medium heat.

- Place in onion, celery, and carrot and cook for 5 minutes. Transfer to the rice bowl.

- Mix in flour, parsley, salt, and pepper. Place in the fridge for 20 minutes. Mold the mixture into cylinder-shaped balls.

- Heat the remaining oil in a skillet over medium heat. Fry the croquettes for 8 minutes, turning occasionally until golden.

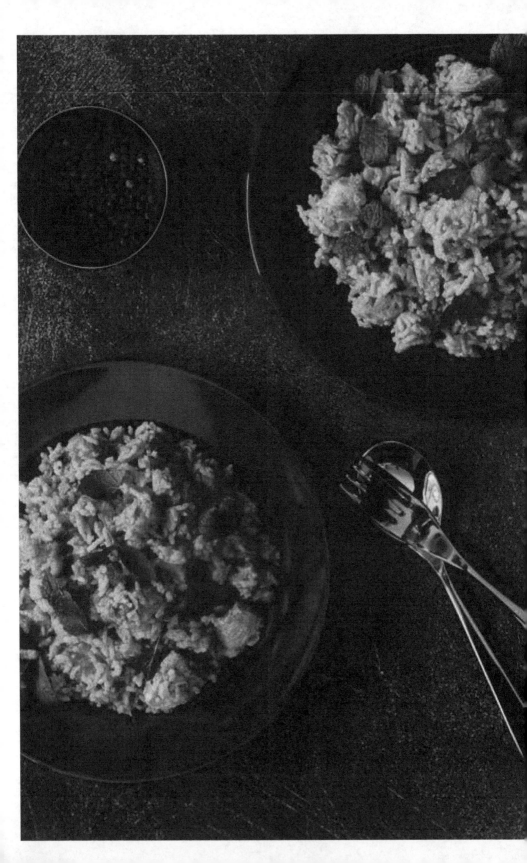

Oregano Chickpeas

6 Servings

Preparation Time: 5 minutes

Ingredients

- 1 tsp olive oil
- 2 tsps dried oregano
- Salt and black pepper to taste
- 1 onion, cut into half-moon slices
- 2 (14.5-oz) cans chickpeas
- ½ cup vegetable broth

Directions

- Heat the oil in a skillet over medium heat. Cook the onion for 3 minutes. Stir in chickpeas, broth, oregano, salt, and pepper.

- Bring to a boil, then lower the heat and simmer for 10 minutes. Serve.

Matcha-Infused Tofu Rice

6 Servings

Preparation Time: 35 minutes

Ingredients

- 4 matcha Tea bags
- 3 green Onions, minced
- 2 cups snow Peas, cut diagonally
- 1 tbsp fresh lemon juice
- 1 tsp grated lemon zest
- Salt and black pepper to taste
- 1 ½ cups brown rice
- 2 tbsps Canola oil
- 8 oz extra-firm tofu, chopped

Directions

- Boil 3 cups of water in a pot. Place in the tea bags and turn the heat off.

- Let sit for 7 minutes. Discard the bags.

- Wash the rice and put it into the tea.

- Cook for 20 minutes over medium heat. Drain and set aside.

- Heat the oil in a skillet over medium heat. Fry the tofu for 5 minutes until golden.

- Stir in green onions and snow peas and cook for another 3 minutes. Mix in lemon juice and lemon zest.

- Place the rice in a serving bowl and mix in the tofu mixture

- . Adjust the seasoning with salt and pepper. Serve right away.

Chinese Fried Rice

6 Servings

Preparation Time: 20 minutes

Ingredients

- 2 tbsps Canola oil
- 3 green onions, minced
- 3 ½ cups cooked brown rice
- 1 cup frozen peas, thawed
- 3 tbsps soy sauce
- 2 tsps dry white wine
- 1 tbsp toasted sesame oil
- 1 onion, chopped
- 1 large carrot, chopped
- 1 head broccoli, cut into florets
- 2 Garlic cloves, minced
- 2 tsps grated fresh ginger

Directions

- Heat the oil in a pan over medium heat.
- Place in onion, carrot, and broccoli, sauté for 5 minutes until tender.
- Add in garlic, ginger, and green onions and sauté for another 3 minutes. Stir in rice, peas, soy sauce, and white wine and cook for 5 minutes.
- Add in sesame oil, toss to combine. Serve right away.

Savory Seitan &Bell Pepper Rice

6 Servings

Preparation Time: 35 minutes

Ingredients

- 2 cups water
- 1 green bell pepper, chopped
- 1 tsp dried basil
- ½ tsp ground fennel seeds
- ¼ tsp crushed red pepper
- Salt and black pepper to taste
- 1 cup long-grain brown rice
- 2 tbsps olive oil
- 1 onion, chopped
- 2 garlic cloves, minced
- 8 oz seitan, chopped

Directions

- Bring water to a boil in a pot.
- Place in rice and lower the heat. Simmer for 20 minutes.
- Heat the oil in a pan over medium heat.
- Cook the onion for 3 minutes.
- Stir in chickpeas, broth, oregano, salt, and pepper.
- Bring to a boil, then lower the heat and simmer for 10 minutes. Serve

Asparagus & Mushrooms with Mashed Potatoes

6 Servings

Preparation Time: 60 minutes

Ingredients

- 5 large portobello mushrooms
- 2 tsps Olive oil
- 2 tsps nutritional yeast
- ½ cup non-dairy milk
- 7 cups asparagus, chopped
- 6 Potatoes chopped
- Sea salt to taste
- 4 Garlic cloves
- 3tsp Coconut oil

Direction

- Placed chopped potatoes in a pot and cover with salted water cook 20 minutes
- Heat oil in a pan sauté garlic
- Once potatoes are ready, drain them and reserve the water
- Now mash them
- Put some hot water, garlic, milk, yeast, and salt
- Preheat your grill, grease the mushrooms
- After grill as asparagus for about 10 minutes, arrange the veggies in a serving platter and serve with mash potatoes

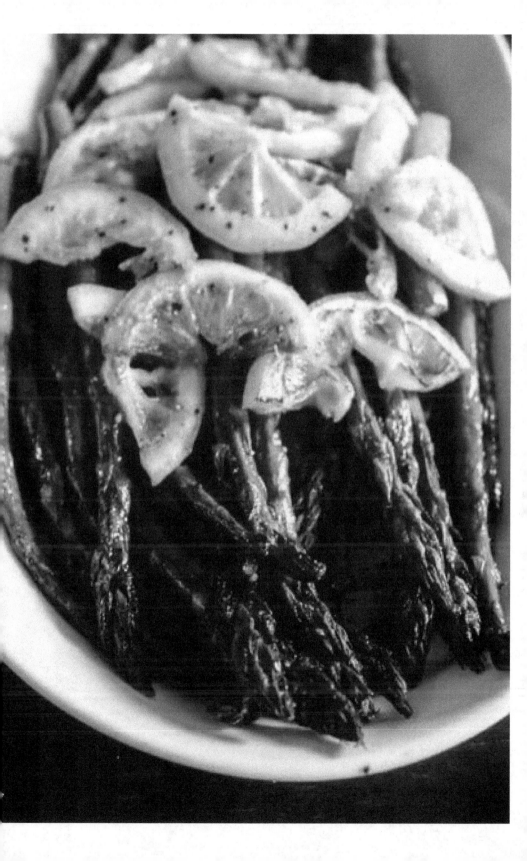

DESSERT

Chocolate Peppermint Mousse

4 Servings

Preparation Time: 10 minutes

Ingredients

- ¼ cup Swerve sugar, divided
- 4 oz cashew cream cheese, softened
- 3 tbsps cocoa powder
- ¾ tsp peppermint extract
- ½ tsp vanilla extract
- 1/3 cup coconut cream

Directions

- Put 2 tablespoons of Swerve sugar, cashew cream cheese, and cocoa powder in a blender.

- Add the peppermint extract, ¼ cup warm water, and process until smooth. In a bowl, whip vanilla extract, coconut cream, and the remaining Swerve sugar using a whisk.

- Fetch out 5-6 tablespoons for garnishing. Fold in the cocoa mixture until thoroughly combined.

- Spoon the mousse into serving cups and chill in the fridge for 30 minutes. Garnish with the reserved whipped cream and serve.

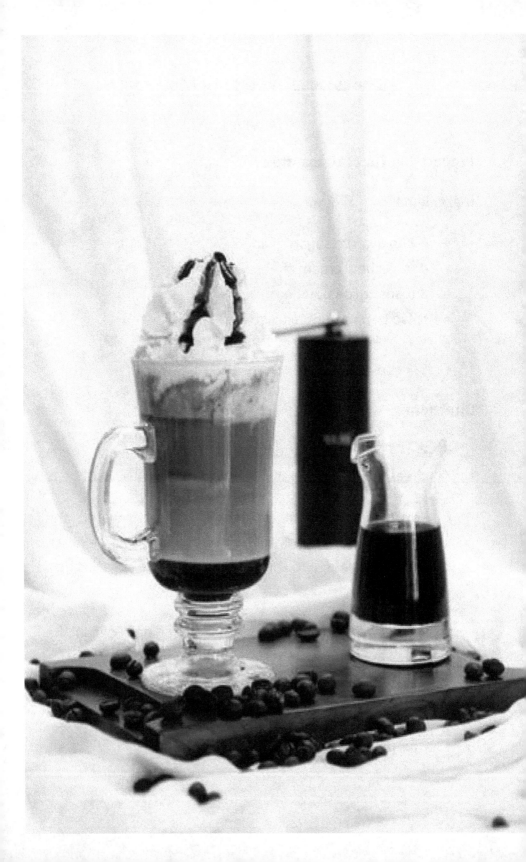

Raspberries Turmeric Panna Cotta

6 Servings

Preparation Time: 10 minutes

Ingredients

- ½ tbsp powdered vegetarian gelatin
- 2 cups coconut cream
- ¼ tsp vanilla extract
- 1 pinch turmeric powder
- 1 tbsp erythritol
- 1 tbsp chopped toasted pecans
- 12 fresh raspberries

Directions

- Mix gelatin and ½ tsp water and allow sitting to dissolve. Pour coconut cream, vanilla extract, turmeric, and erythritol into a saucepan and bring to a boil over medium heat, then simmer for 2 minutes. Turn the heat off.

- Stir in the gelatin until dissolved. Pour the mixture into 6 glasses, cover with plastic wrap, and refrigerate for 2 hours or more.

- Top with the pecans and raspberries and serve.

Banana Pudding

4 Servings

Preparation Time: 30 minutes

Ingredients

- 1 cup unsweetened almond milk
- 2 cups cashew cream
- ¾ cup + 1 tbsp pure date sugar
- ¼ tsp salt
- 3 tbsps cornstarch
- 2 tbsps plant butter, cut into 4 pieces
- 1 tsp vanilla extract
- 2 banana, sliced

Directions

- In a medium pot, mix almond milk, cashew cream, date sugar, and salt.

- Cook over medium heat until slightly thickened, 10-15 minutes. Stir in the cornstarch, plant butter, vanilla extract, and banana extract.

- Cook further for 1 to 2 minutes or until the pudding thickens.

- Dish the pudding into 4 serving bowls and chill in the refrigerator for at least 1 hour.

- To serve, top with the bananas and enjoy!

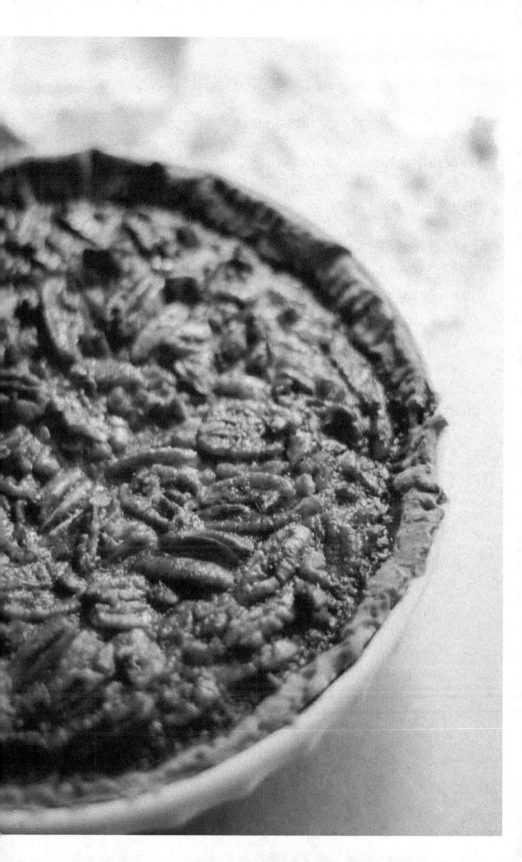

Baked Apples Filled with Nuts

4 Servings

Preparation Time: 35 minutes

Ingredients for 4 servings

- 4 gala apples
- 3 tbsps pure maple syrup
- 4 tbsps almond flour
- 6 tbsps pure date sugar
- 6 tbsps plant butter, cold and cubed
- 1 cup chopped mixed nuts

Directions

- Preheat the oven the 400 F.

- Slice off the top of the apples and use a melon baller or spoon to scoop out the cores of the apples.

- In a bowl, mix the maple syrup, almond flour, date sugar, butter, and nuts. Spoon the mixture into the apples and then bake in the oven for 25 minutes or until the nuts are golden brown on top and the apples soft.

- Remove the apples from the oven, allow cooling, and serve.

Mint Ice Cream

4 Servings

Preparation Time: 10 minutes

Ingredients

- 2 avocados, pitted
- 1 ¼ cups coconut cream
- ½ tsp vanilla extract
- 2 tbsps erythritol
- 2 tsps chopped mint leaves

Directions

- Into a blender, spoon the avocado pulps, pour in the coconut cream, vanilla extract, erythritol, and mint leaves.

- Process until smooth. Pour the mixture into your ice cream maker and freeze according to the manufacturer's instructions.

- When ready, remove and scoop the ice cream into bowls. Serve.

Cardamom Coconut Fat Bombs

6 Servings

Preparation Time: 10 minutes

Ingredients

- ½ cup grated coconut
- 3 oz plant butter, softened
- ¼ tsp green cardamom powder
- ½ tsp vanilla extract
- ¼ tsp cinnamon powder

Directions

- Pour the grated coconut into a skillet and roast until lightly brown. Set aside to cool.

- In a bowl, combine butter, half of the coconut, cardamom, vanilla, and cinnamon.

- Form balls from the mixture and roll each one in the remaining coconut.

- Refrigerate until ready to serve.

CPSIA information can be obtained
at www.ICGtesting.com
Printed in the USA
BVHW091213130521
607267BV00011B/1368